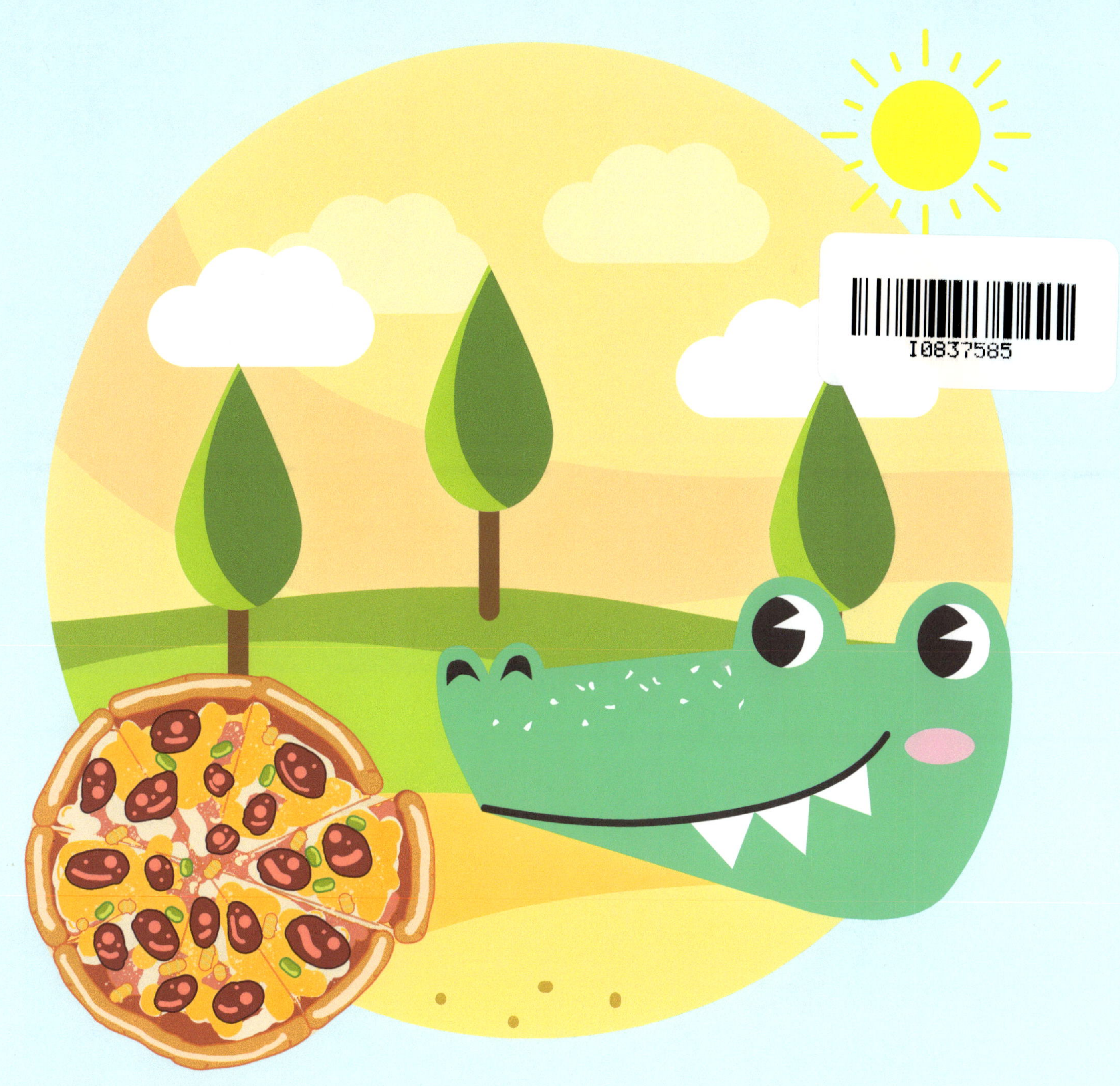

George the croc was a happy dude,
He loved to play and eat his food,
George loved pizza for his tea,
His favourite topping was pepperoni.

1

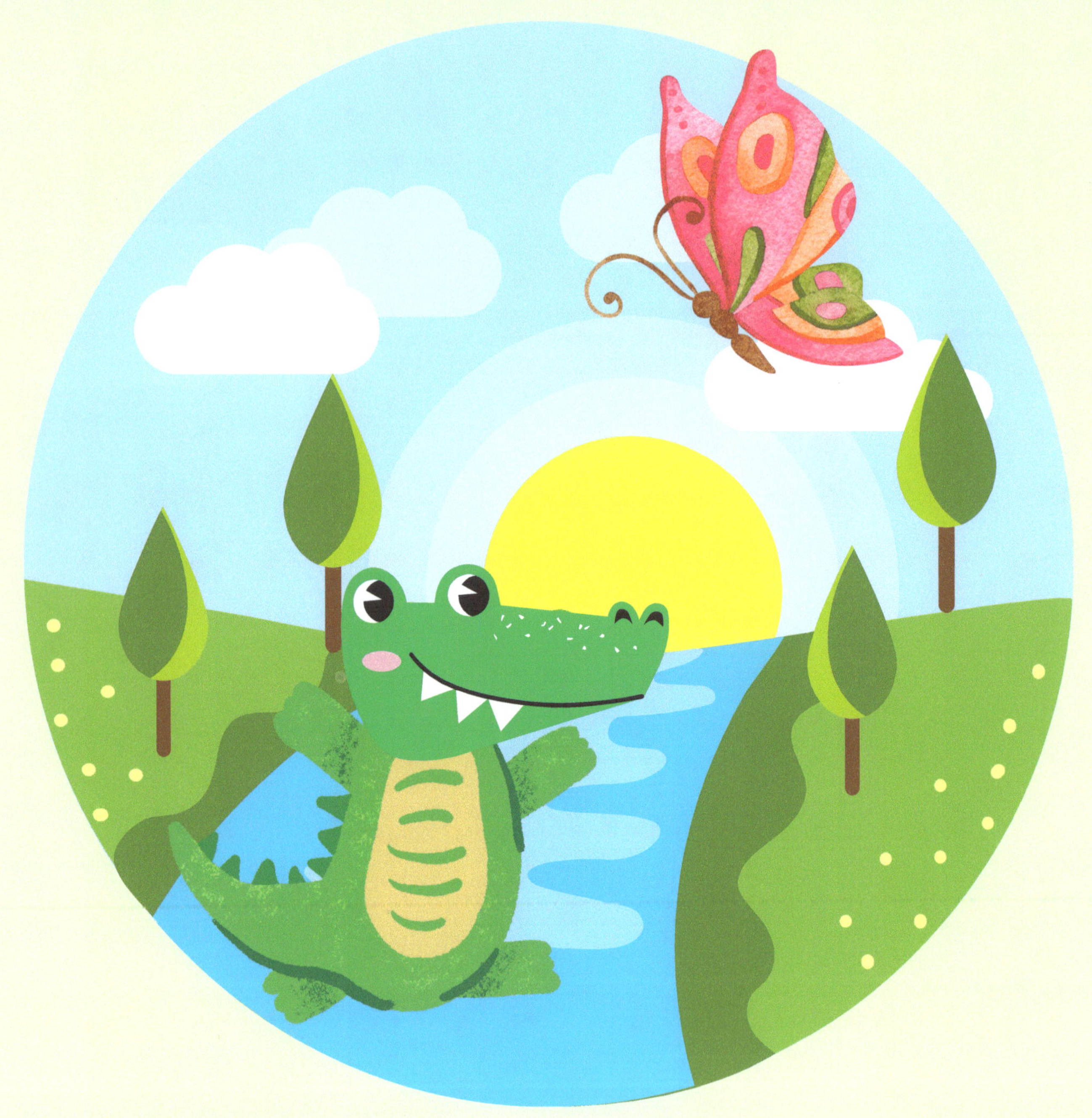

George had big teeth but he was not scary,
He loved to play with his best friend Mary,
Mary was a gentle butterfly,
She knew something was different about George's eyes.

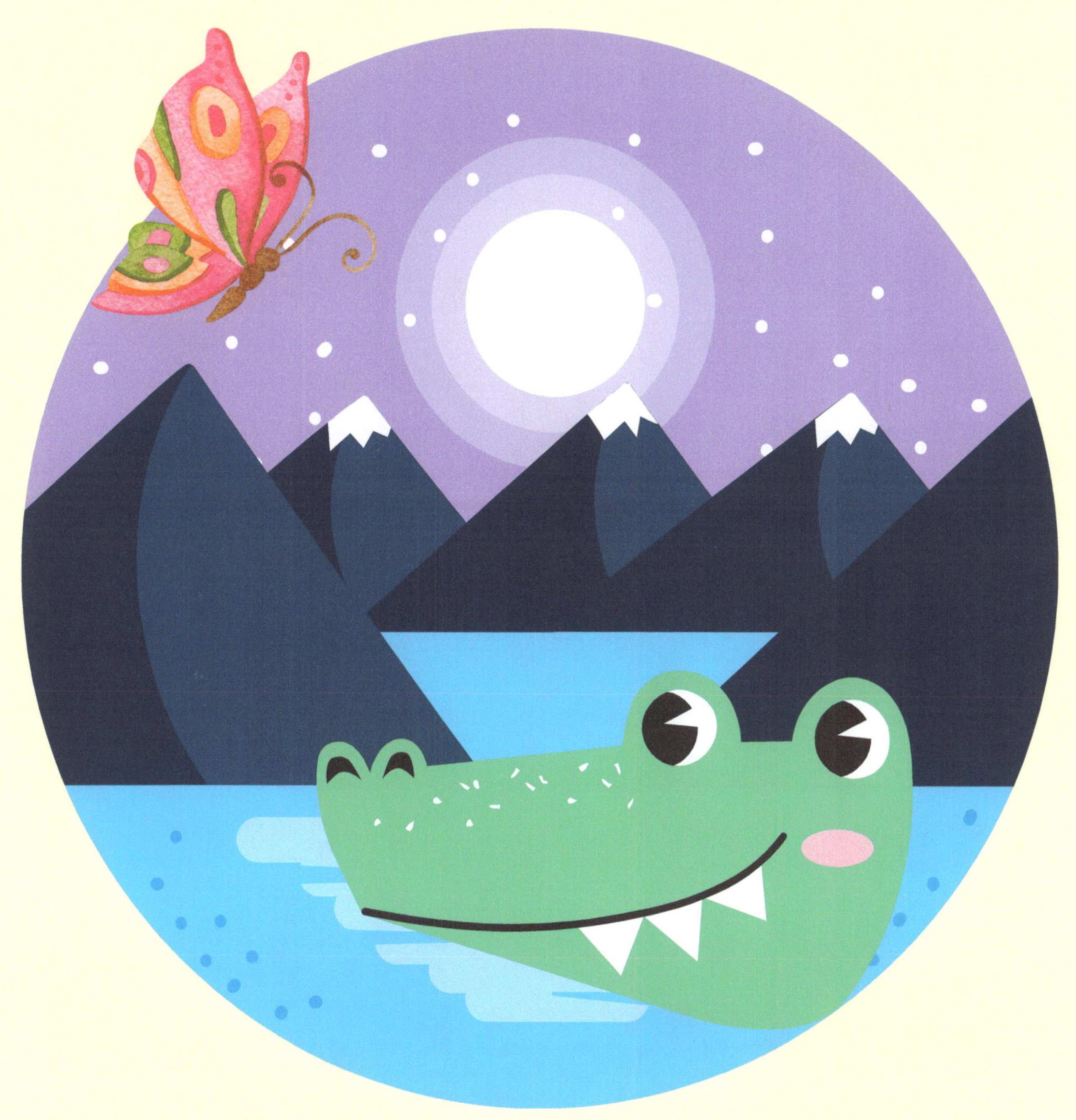

As when the sun came out to play,
George wished that it would go away.
George sometimes said the light was bright,
He seemed to prefer to play at night.

3

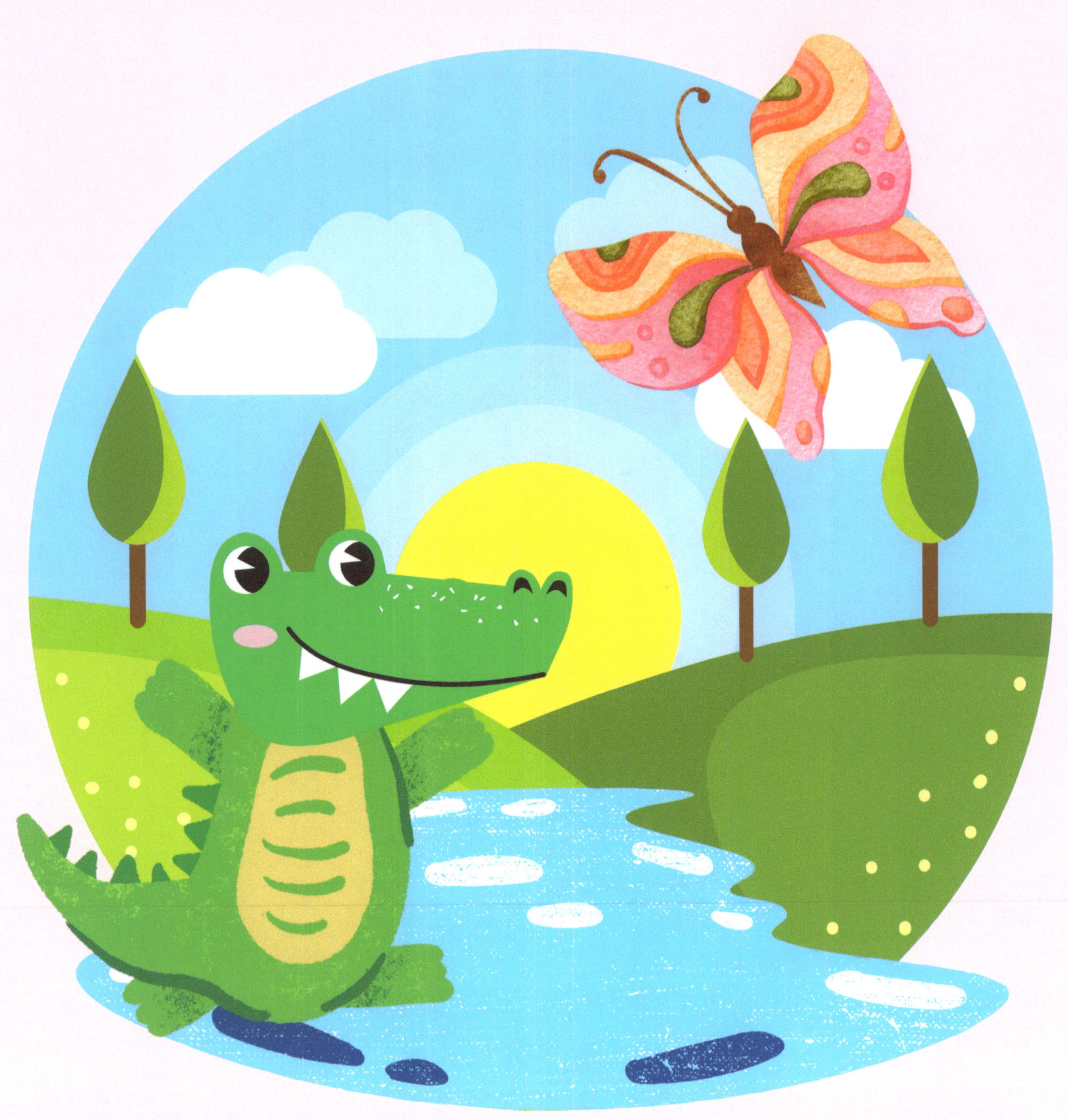

Mary noticed George's eyes would shake,
They shimmered and danced like the sun
on the lake,
George saw his reflection and did declare,
"My eyes are wobbling everywhere!"

4

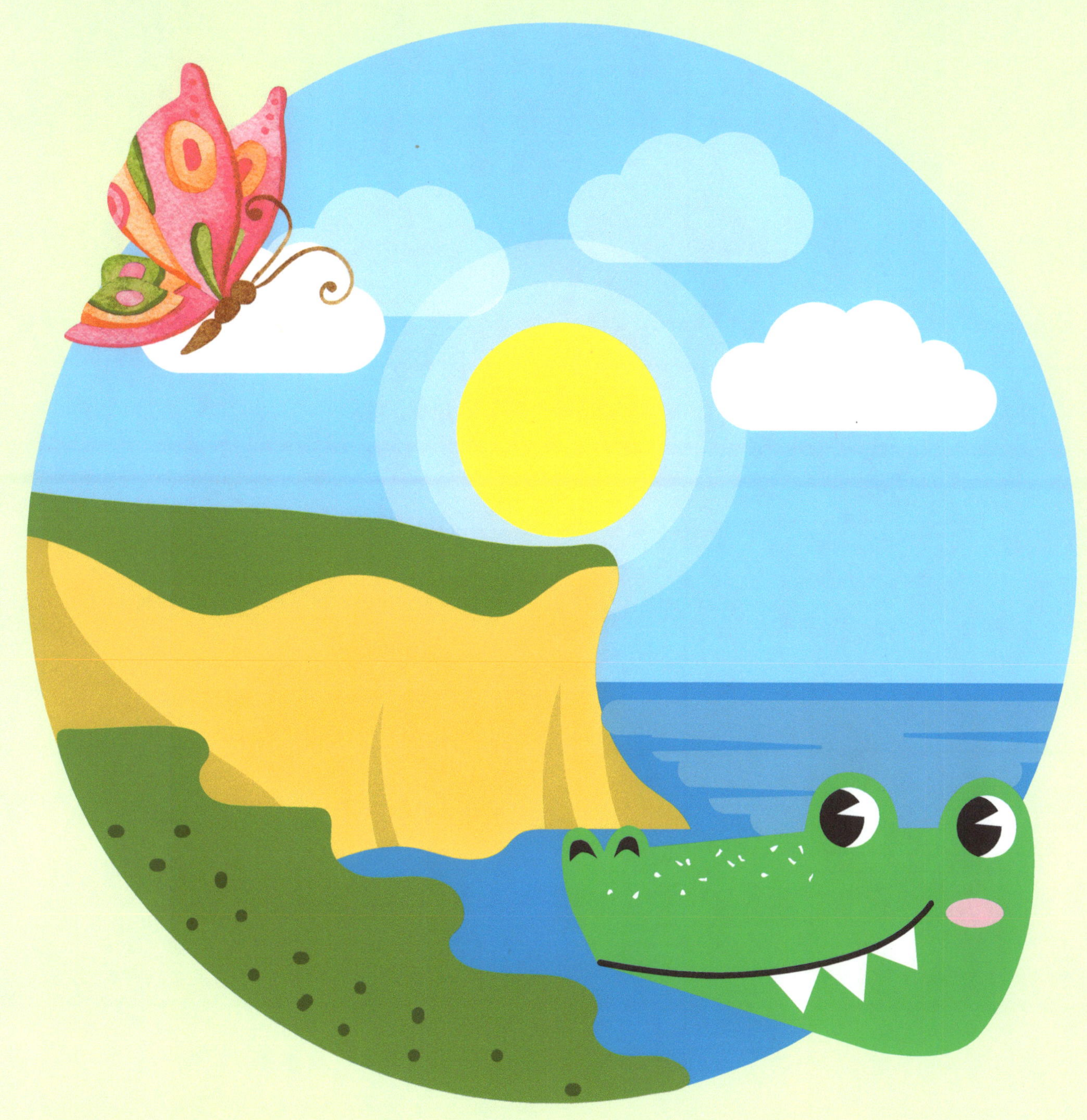

George sometimes bumped into the wall,
He sometimes tripped and he would fall,
He said the beach looked blurry one day,
His vision problems seemed here to stay.

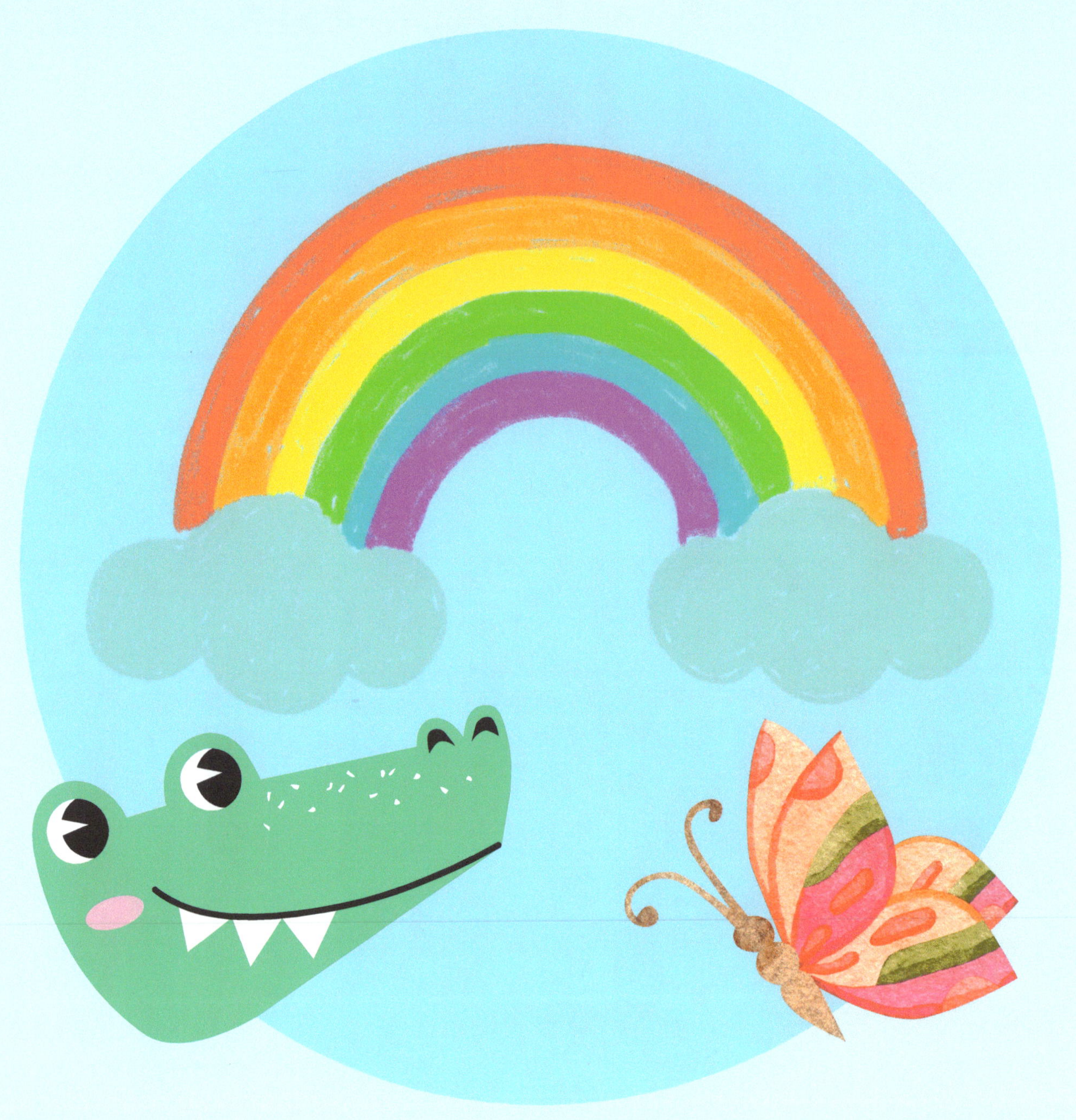

One day a rainbow was in the sky,
So many colours to identify,
George said "this rainbow is in black and white,"
But Mary said "that is not quite right."

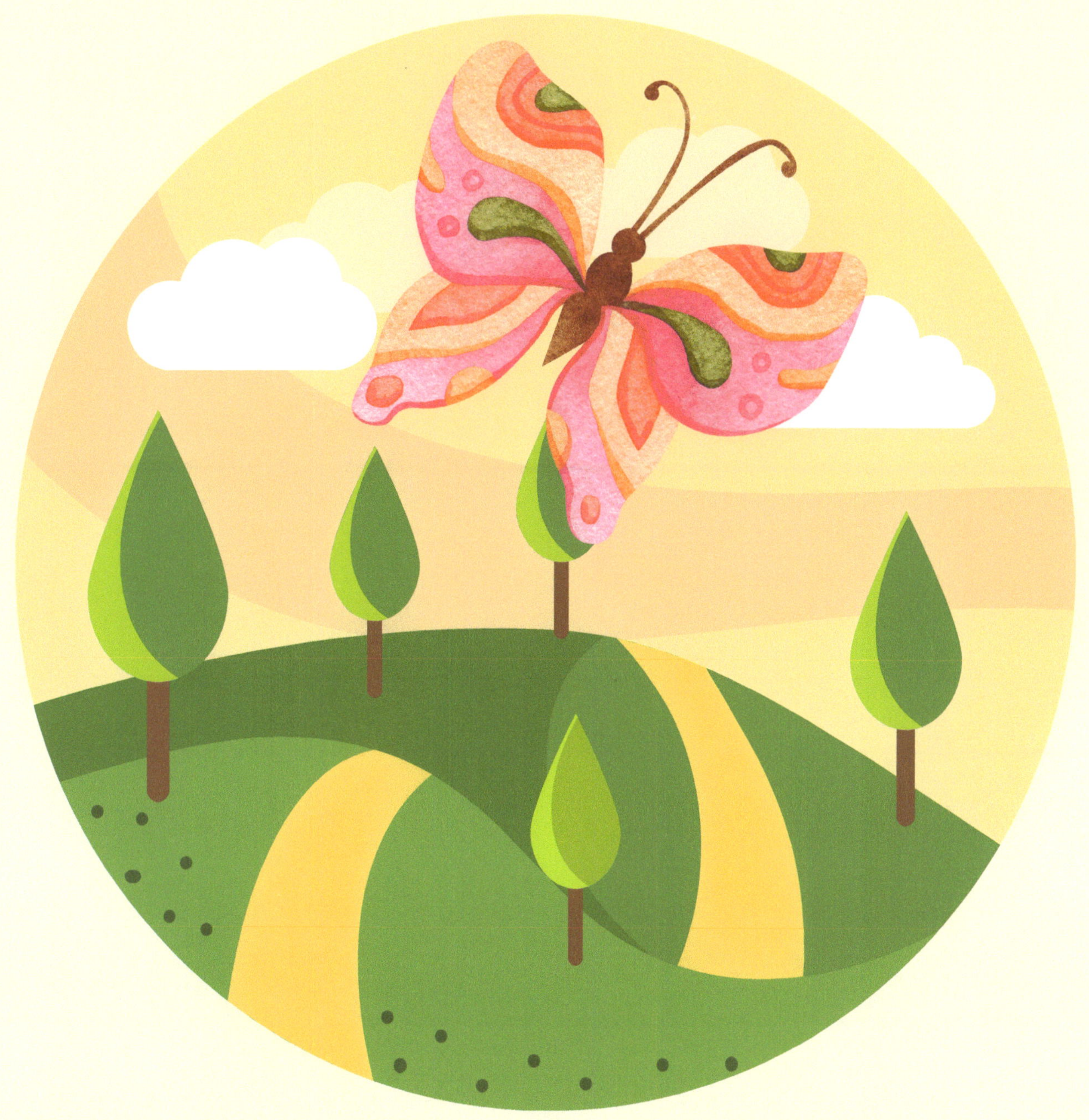

Mary was worried, so later that day,
She flew to get help from far away,
She knew an eye doctor could help them out,
So she asked Doctor Bear to come around.

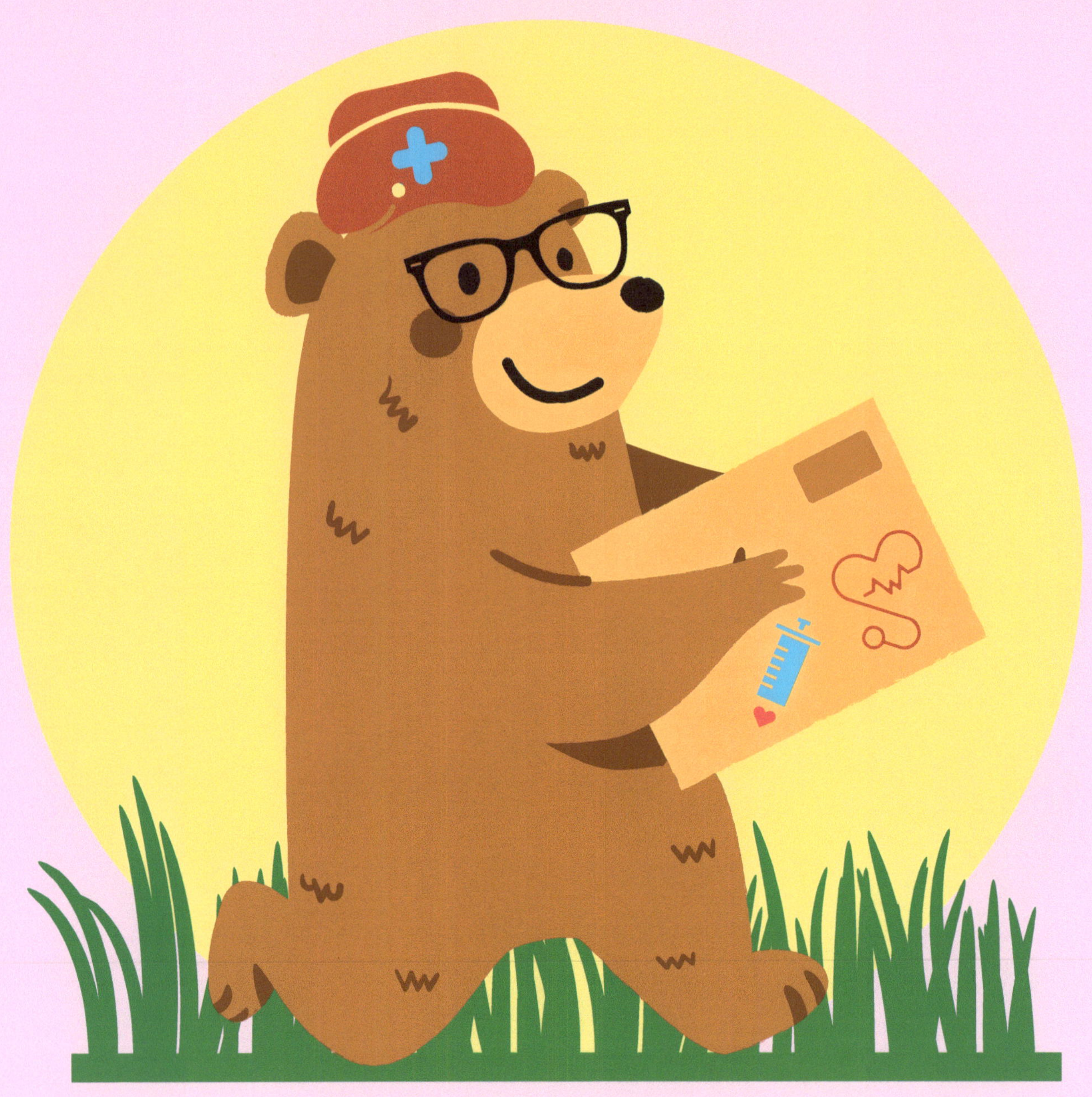

Doctor Bear was an opthamologist too,
This means he checks eyes and sees what they can do,
If something was wrong then he would find out,
Eye tests can show things without a doubt.

8

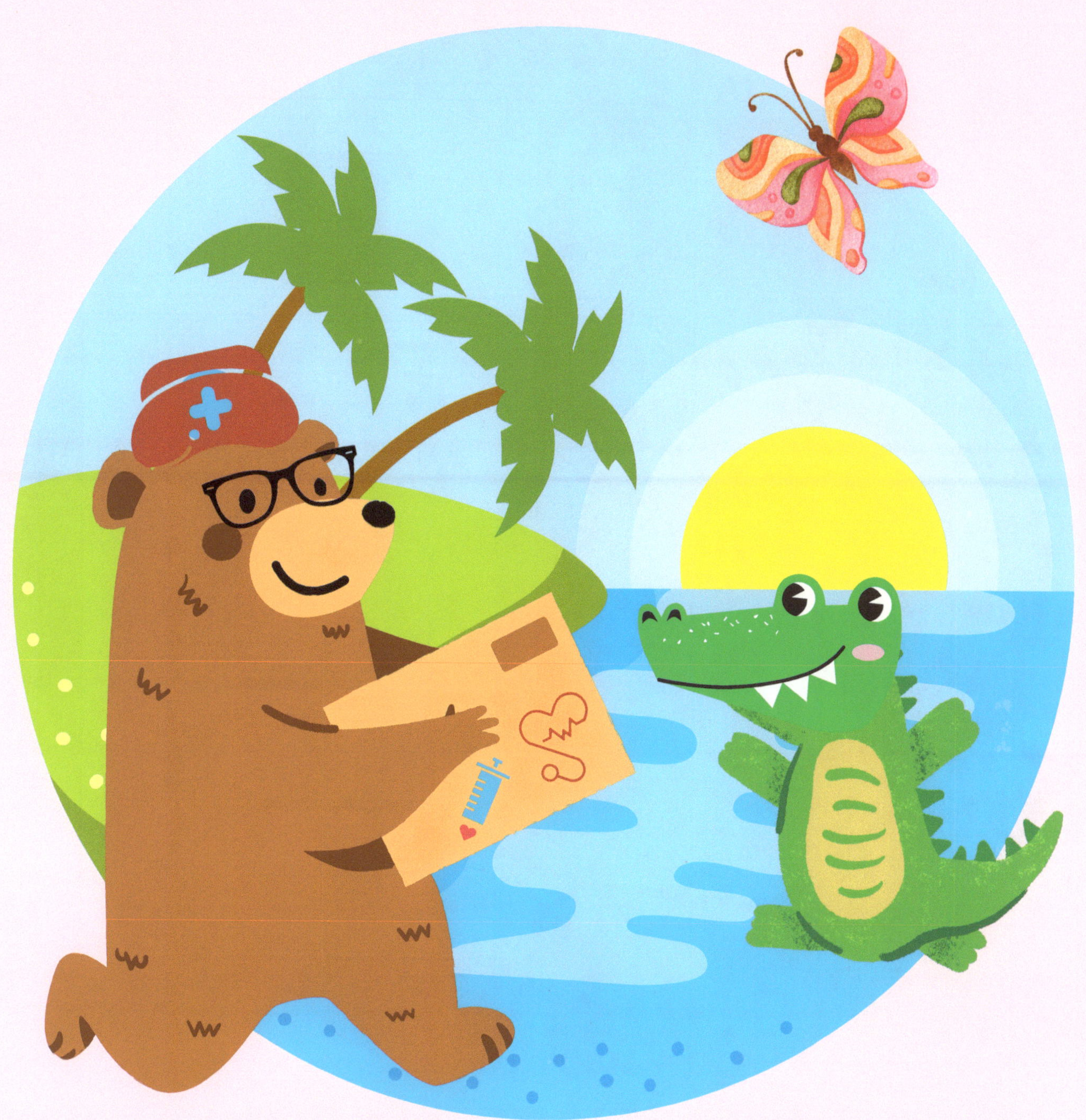

Doctor Bear came to check George's eyes,
He said "George, I have a big surprise,
You have Achromatopsia and Nystagmus too,
But don't worry George there's lots we can do".

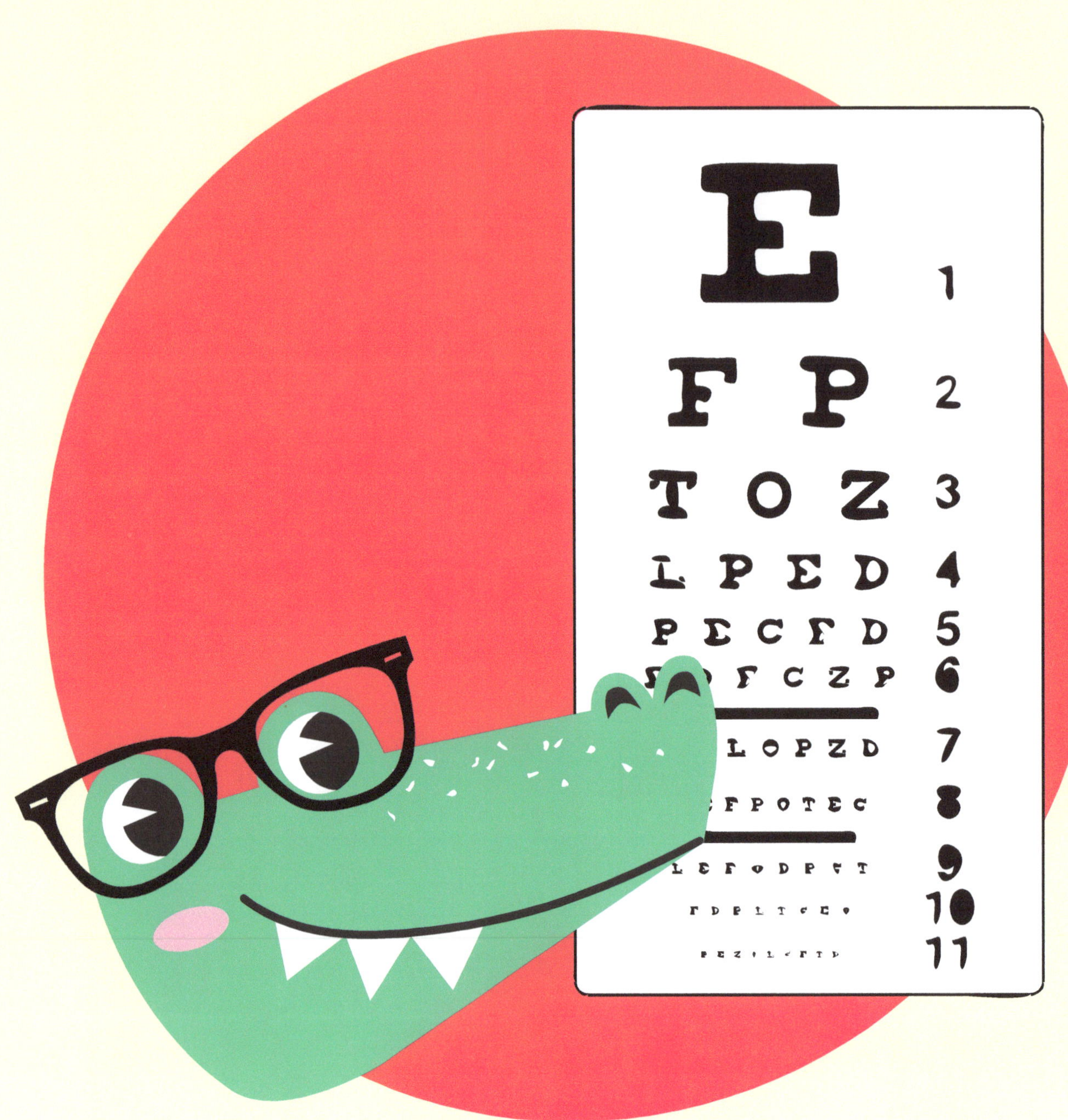

"First let us do an eye test to check your sight,
It is really easy there is no wrong or right,
Just let me know what letters you see,
Then we will know what your eye prescription
should be."

10

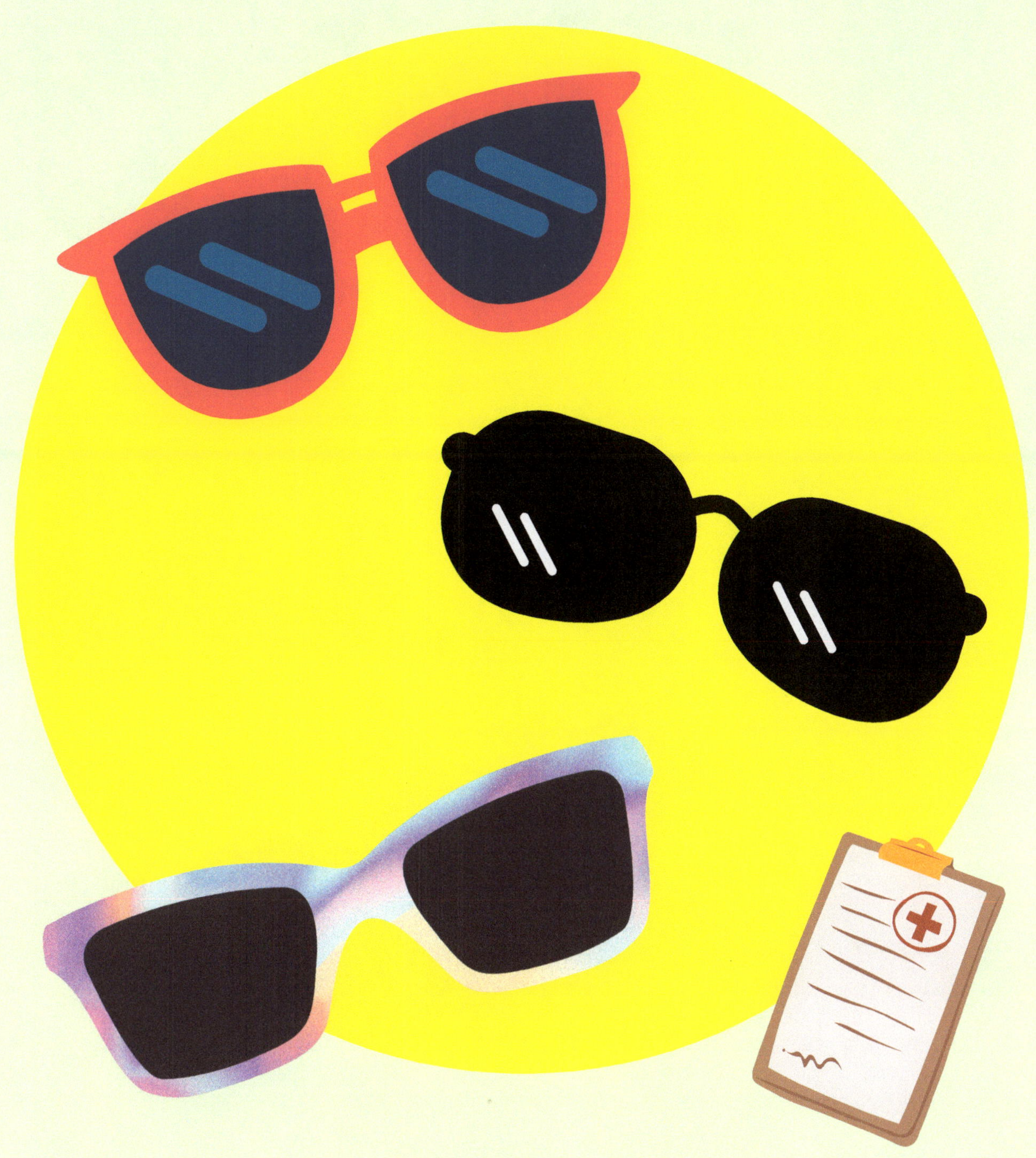

"Next you can pick some cool frames with me,
They are just like sunglasses to help you see,
The dark tint protects your eyes from the light,
These glasses will really enhance your sight."

11

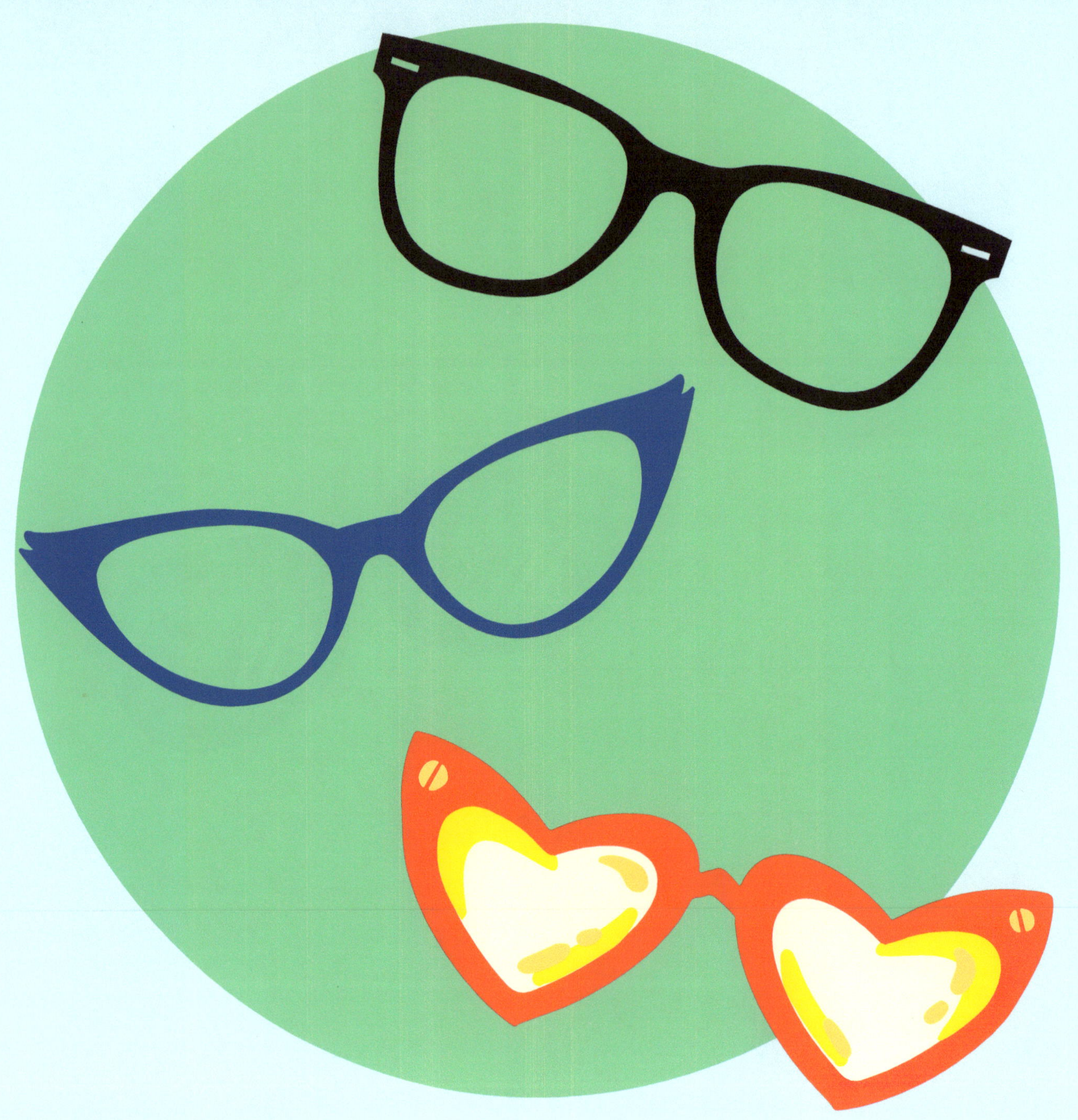

"You can have a pair with a lighter tint too,
Sometimes when indoors these ones will do,
You will soon figure out which pair feels right,
You can vary them based on the day and
night."

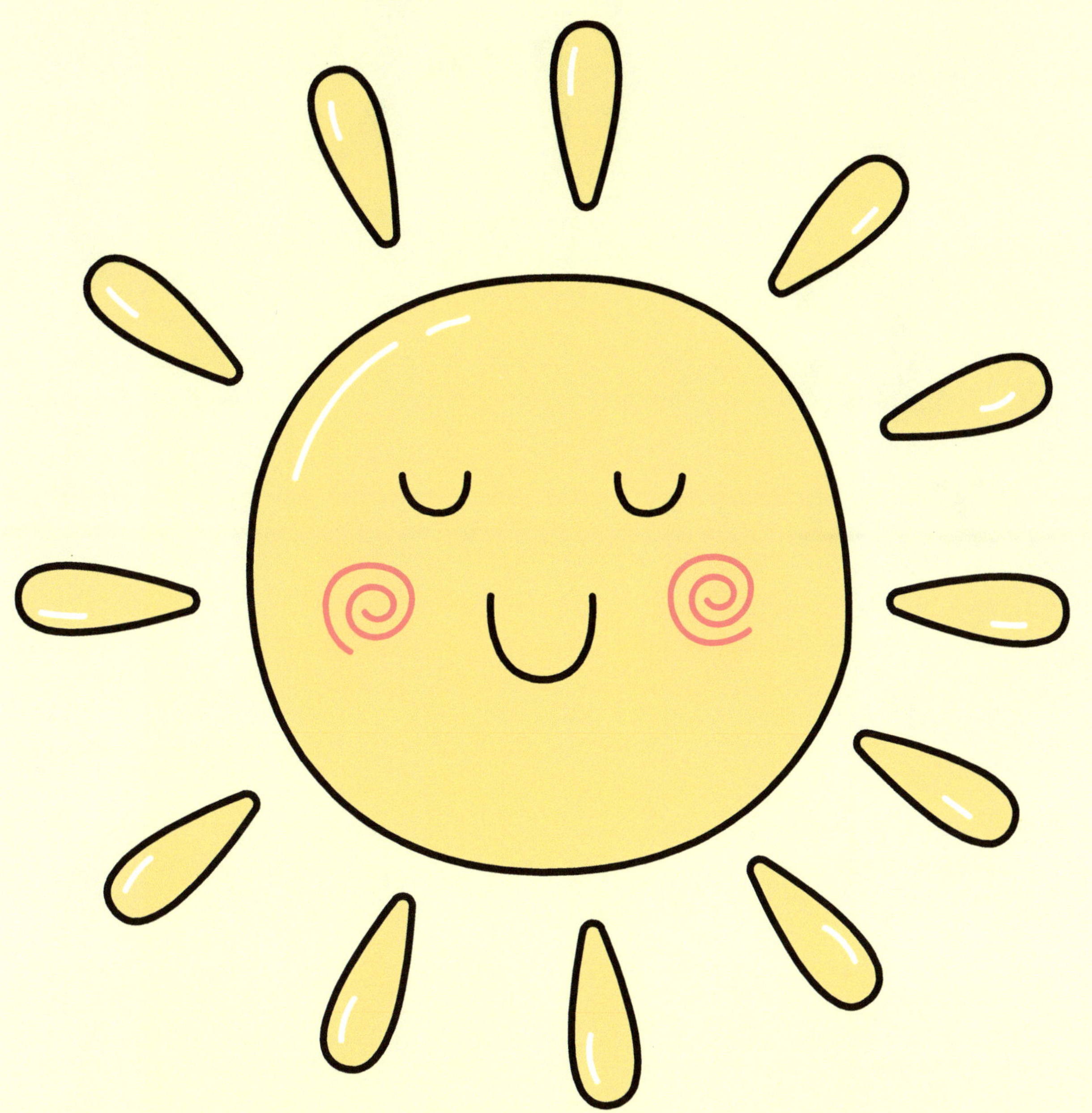

"But now you can play out in the daytime too,
The sun will feel much safer for you,
You will see more shapes and faces as well,
You can play in the lake, it will be swell!"

13

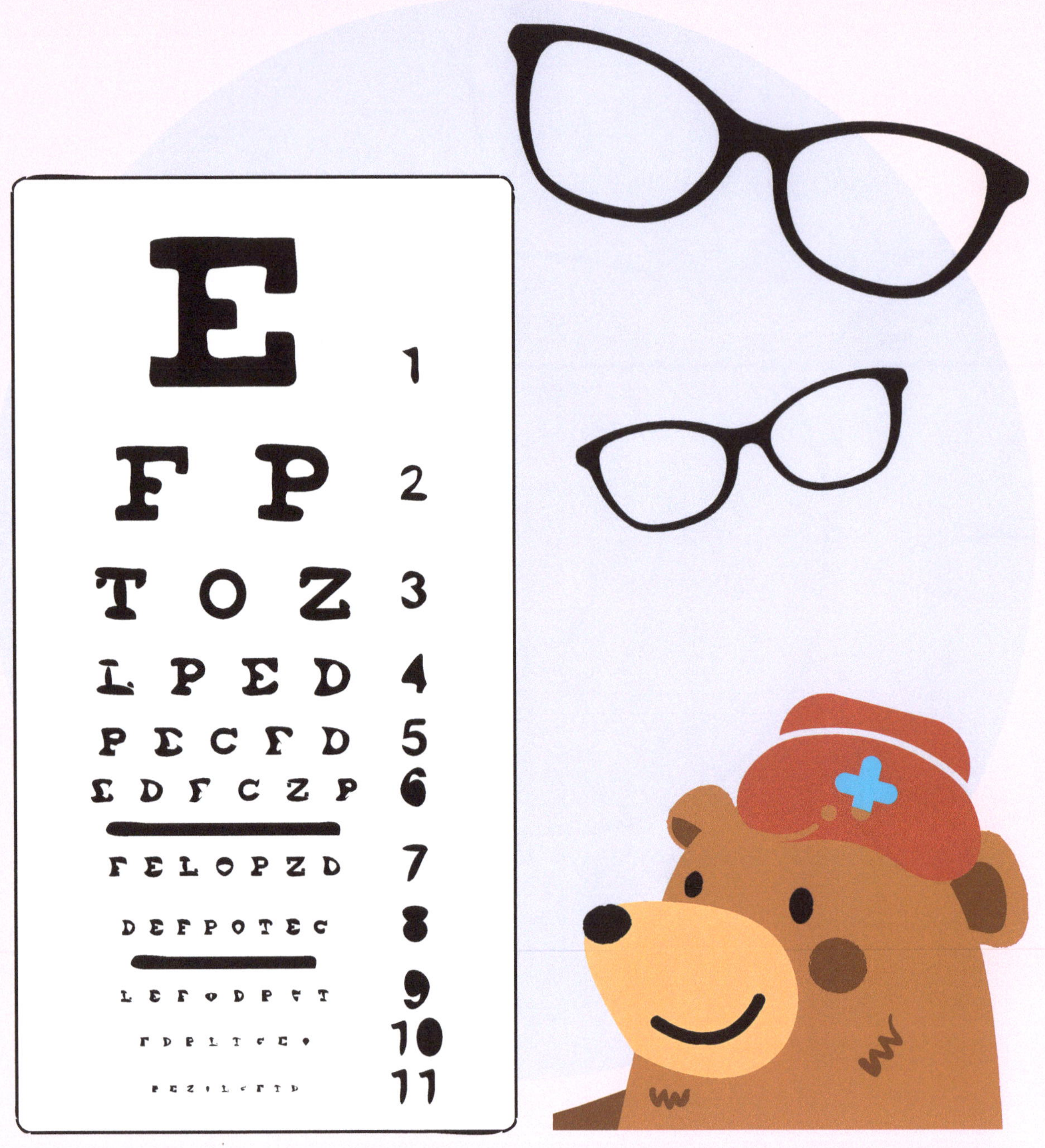

"I will see you for an eye test once a year,
It is easy and simple so have no fear,
I will help you learn just what to do,
When your vision is bothering you."

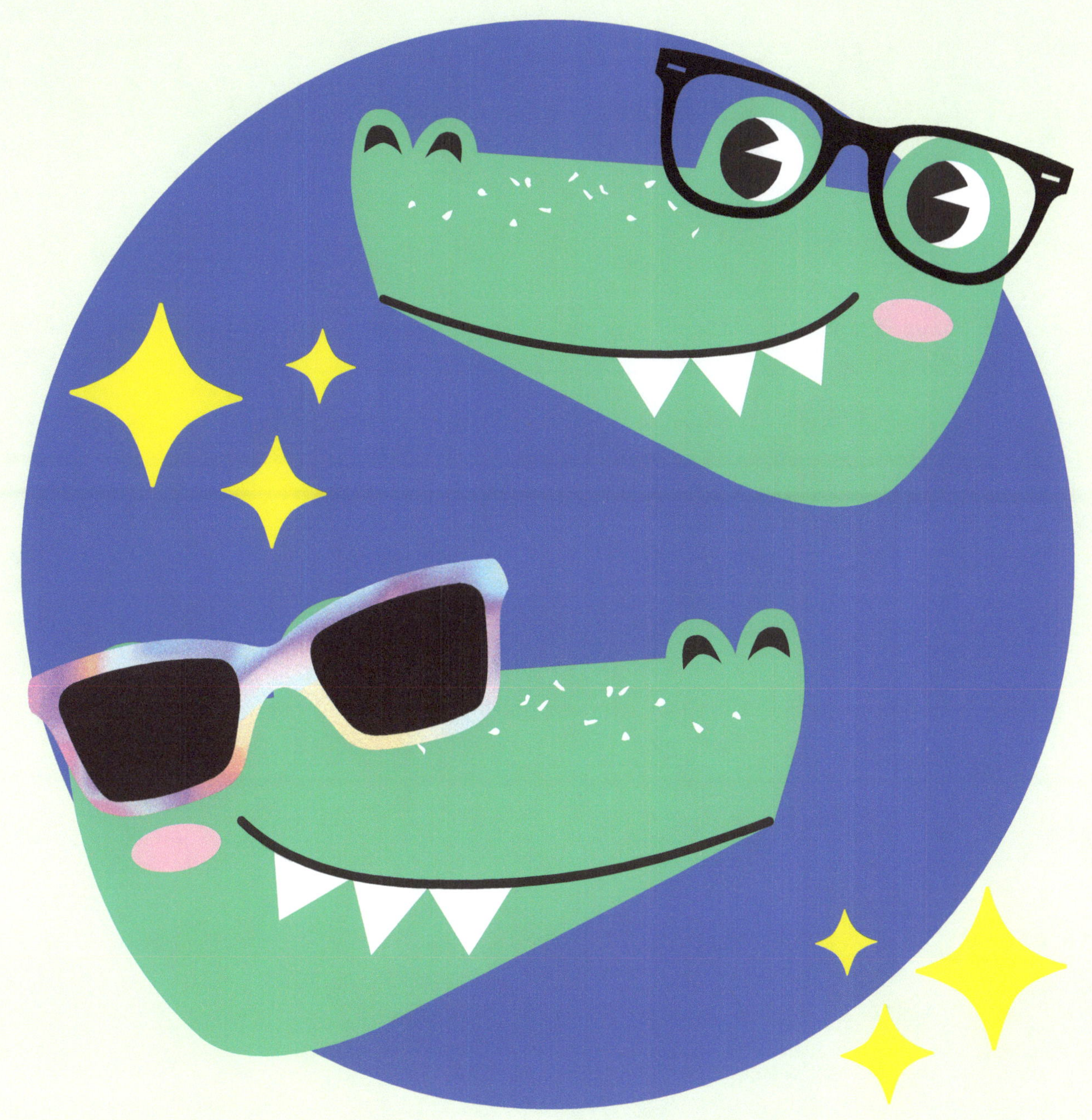

George felt quite sad but glasses were cool,
He would wear them all day and even at school,
He picked some frames that looked quite jazzy,
He felt like a cool croc and rather snazzy!

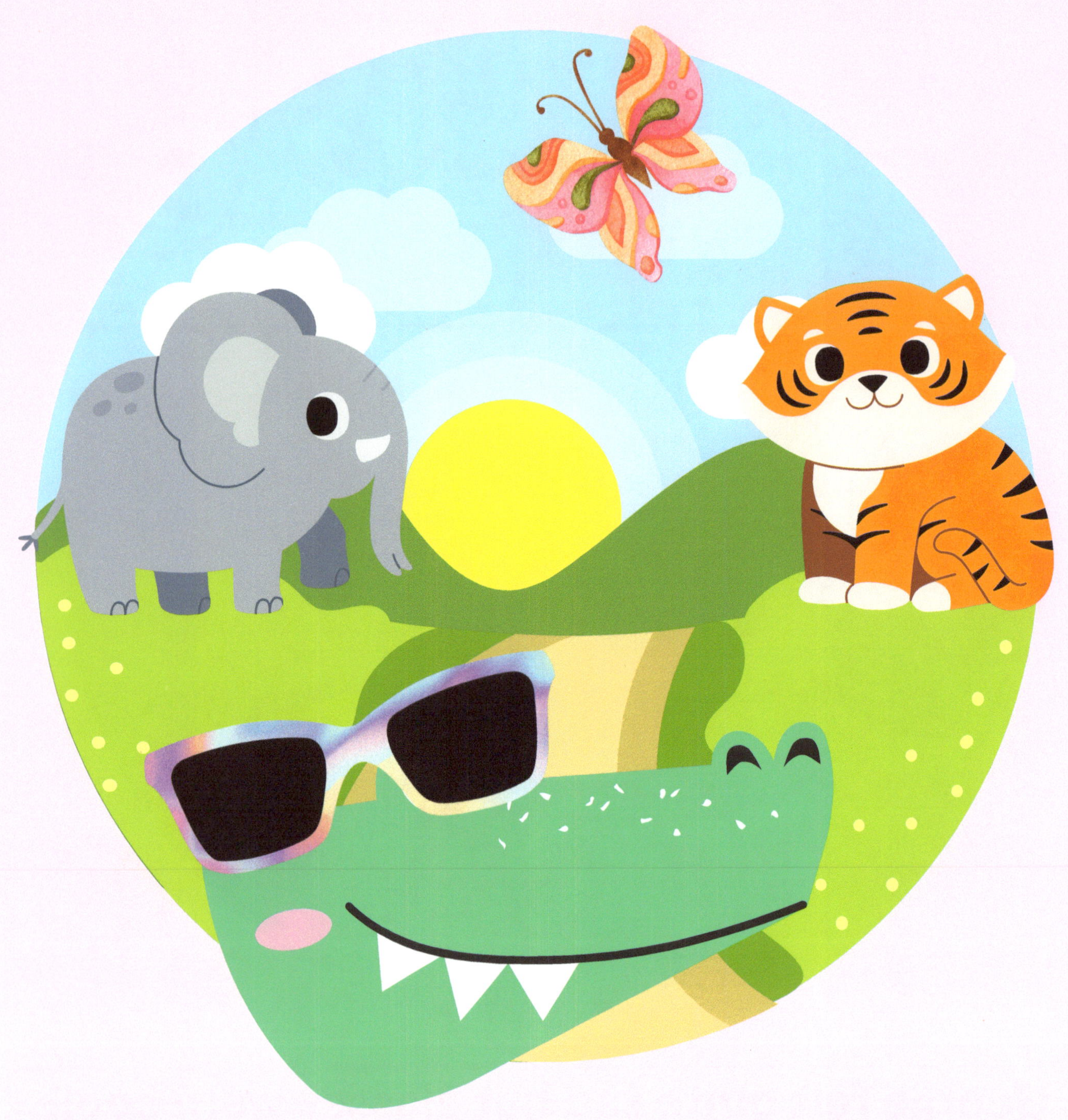

Back at the lake, George went to school,
His friends said "wow, you look so cool!"
George was as confident as could be,
His new glasses were helping him to see.

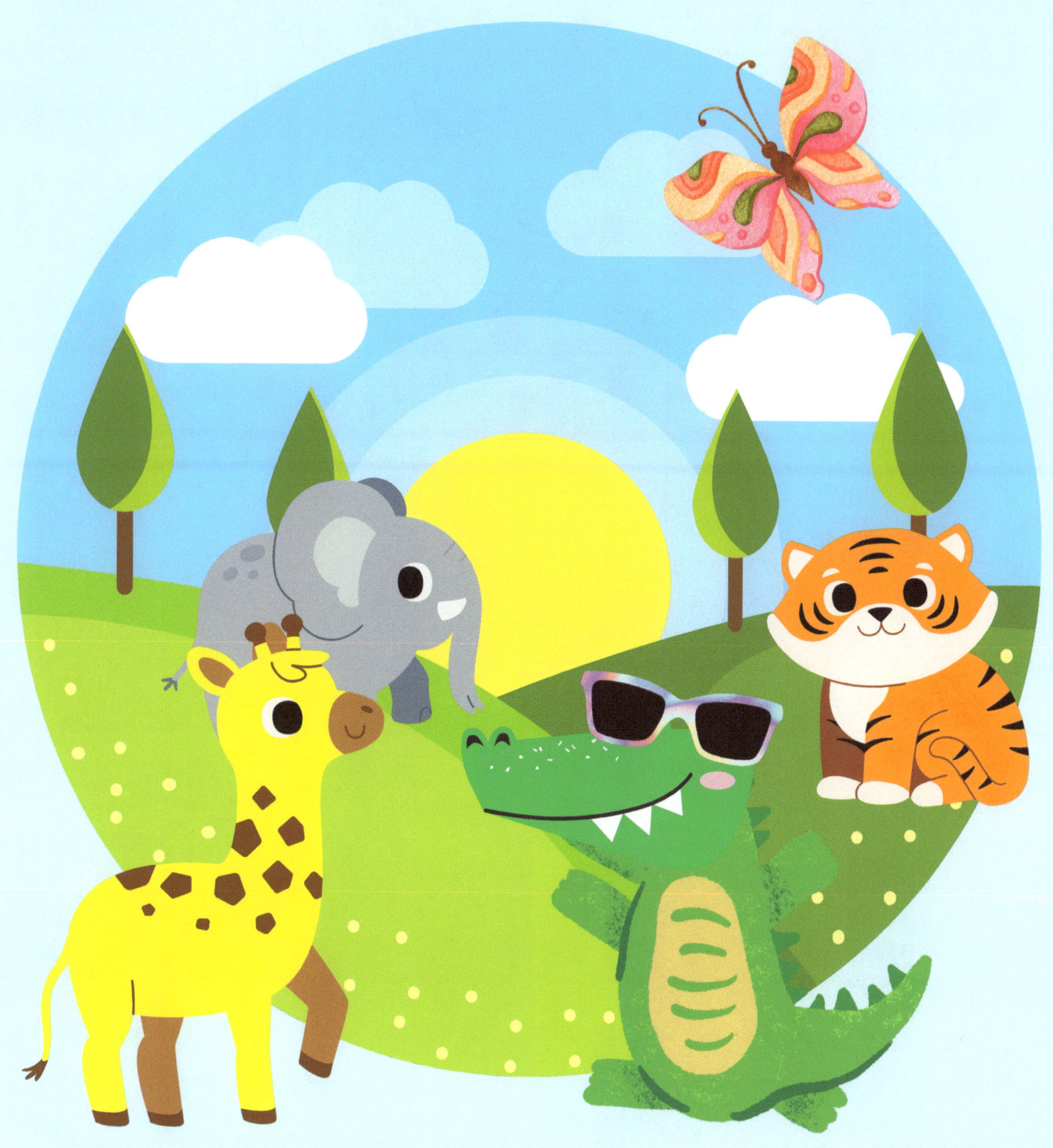

Although George saw in black and white,
With his friends he felt alright,
When he went to play outdoors,
His friends were always there for support.

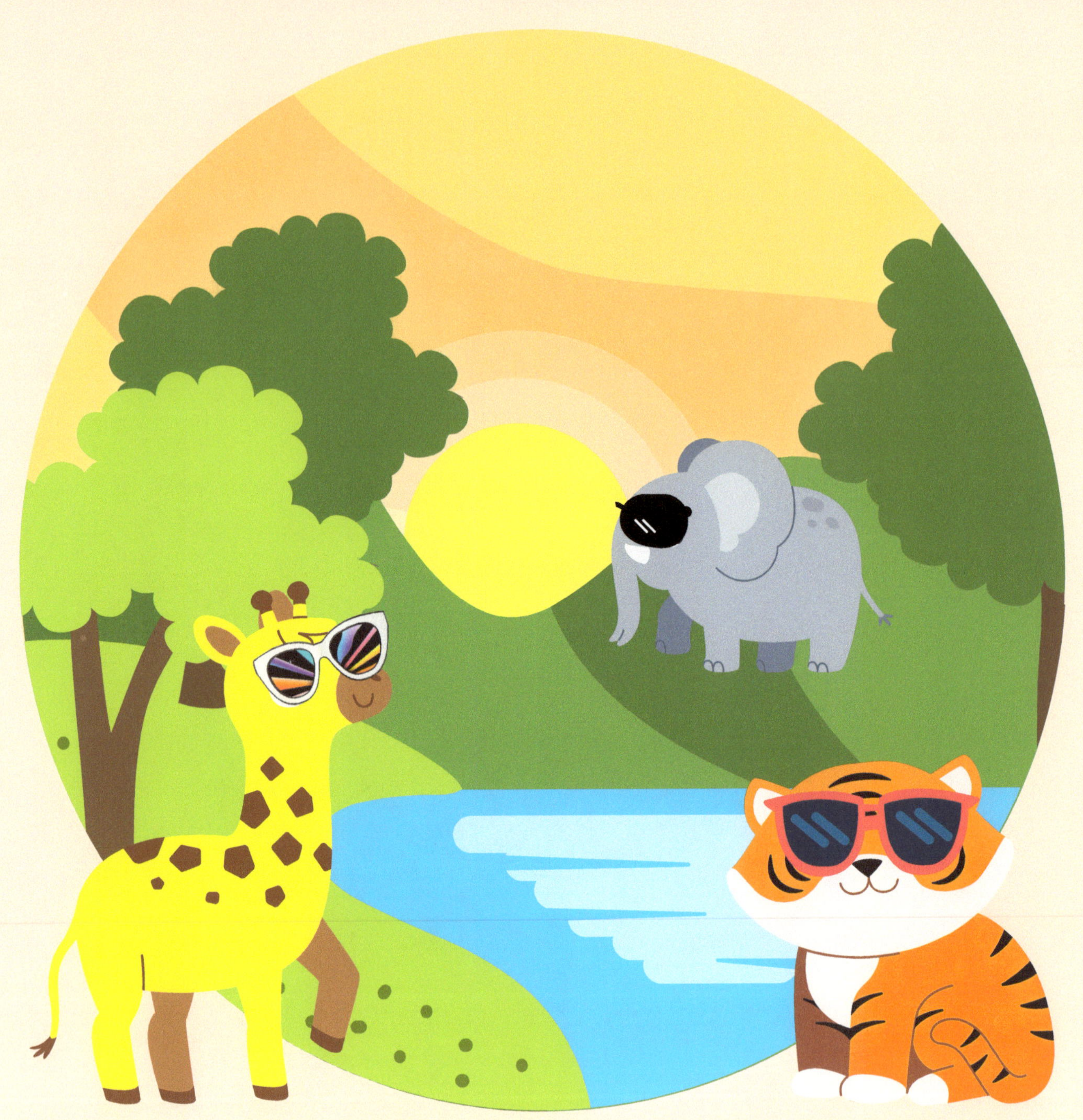

George loved it when the summer came,
His friends wore sunglasses and looked the same,
No-one treated George any differently,
Just because of the way he could see.

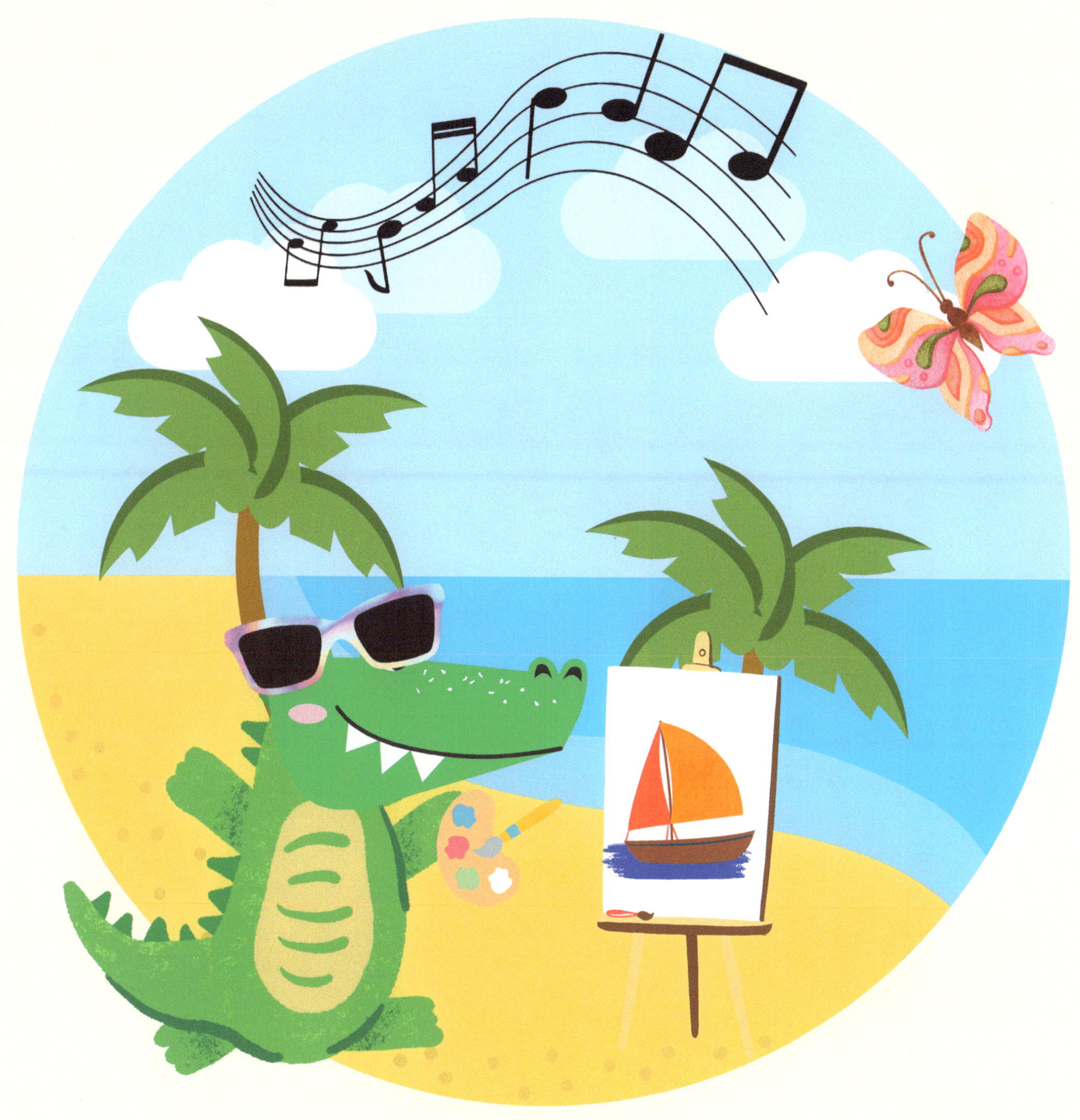

George plays piano and loves to paint,
With his new glasses he feels just great!
He has even learnt to ride his bike,
He loves to run and climb and hike!

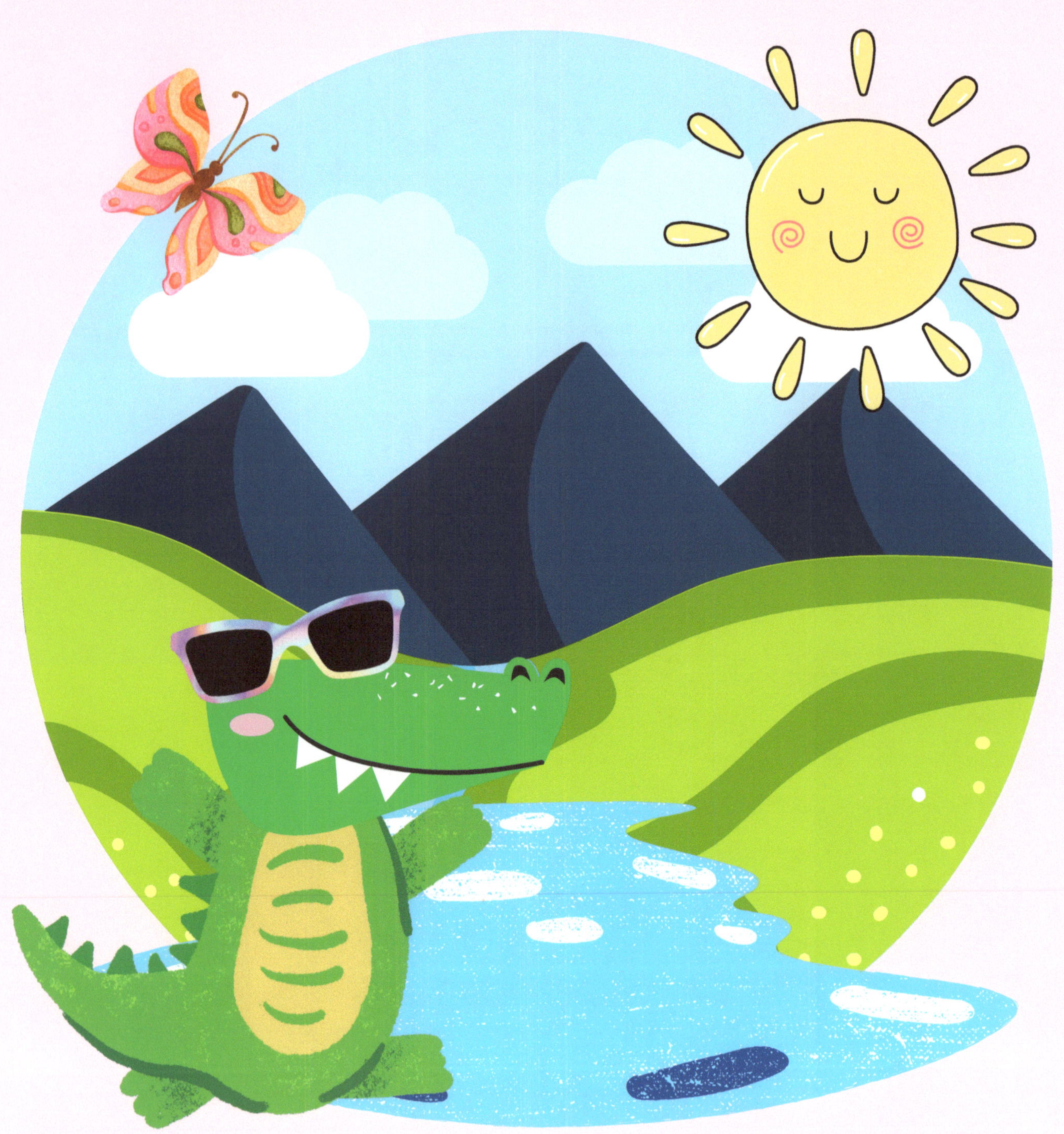

George's eyes still wobble to and fro,
This will keep happening as he grows,
His shimmering eyes will dance all day,
But George will cope in his own way.

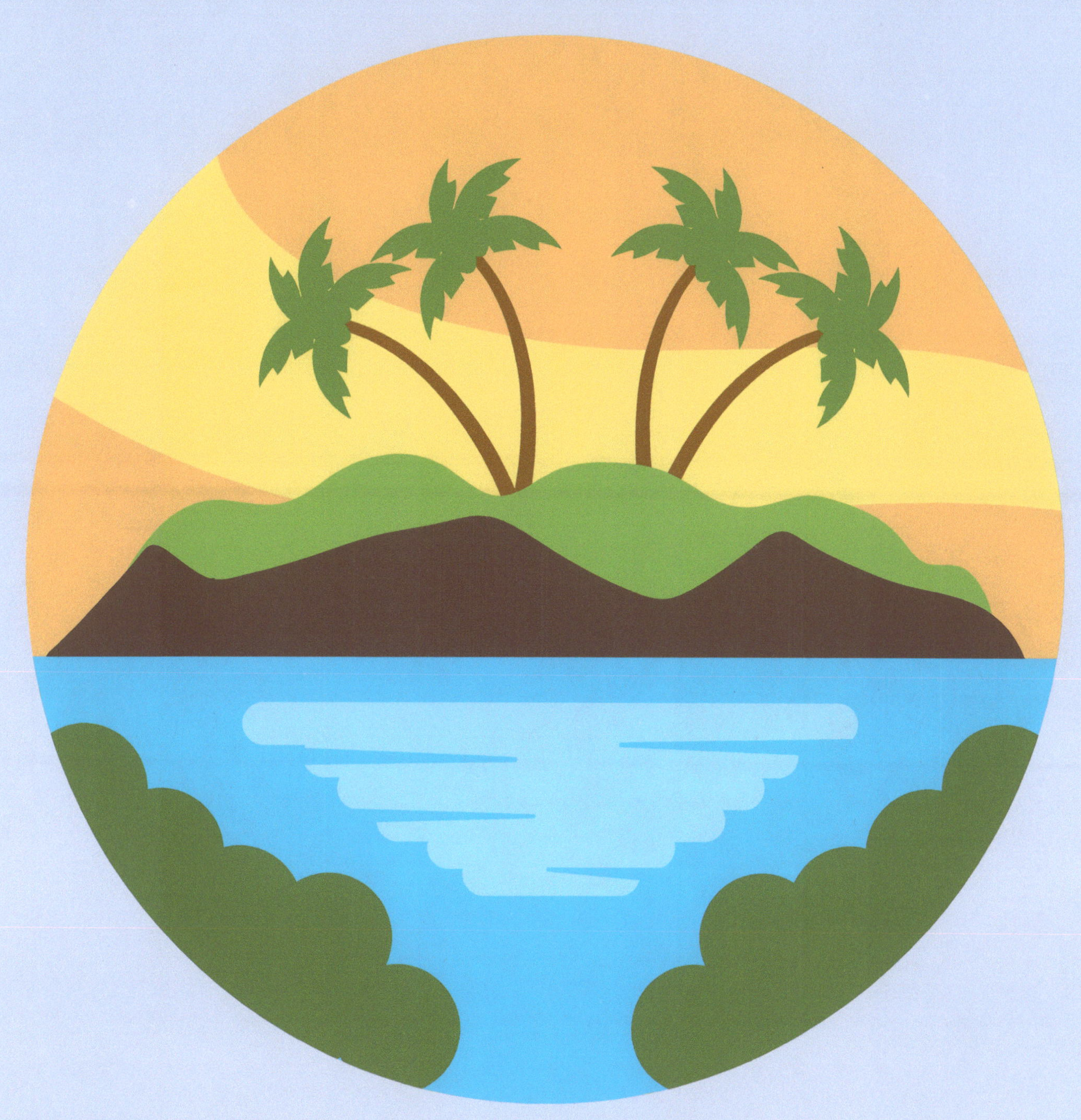

If you have Achromatopsia too,
Your eyes are special just like you,
Rest assurred it will be okay,
You will find new ways to cope each day.

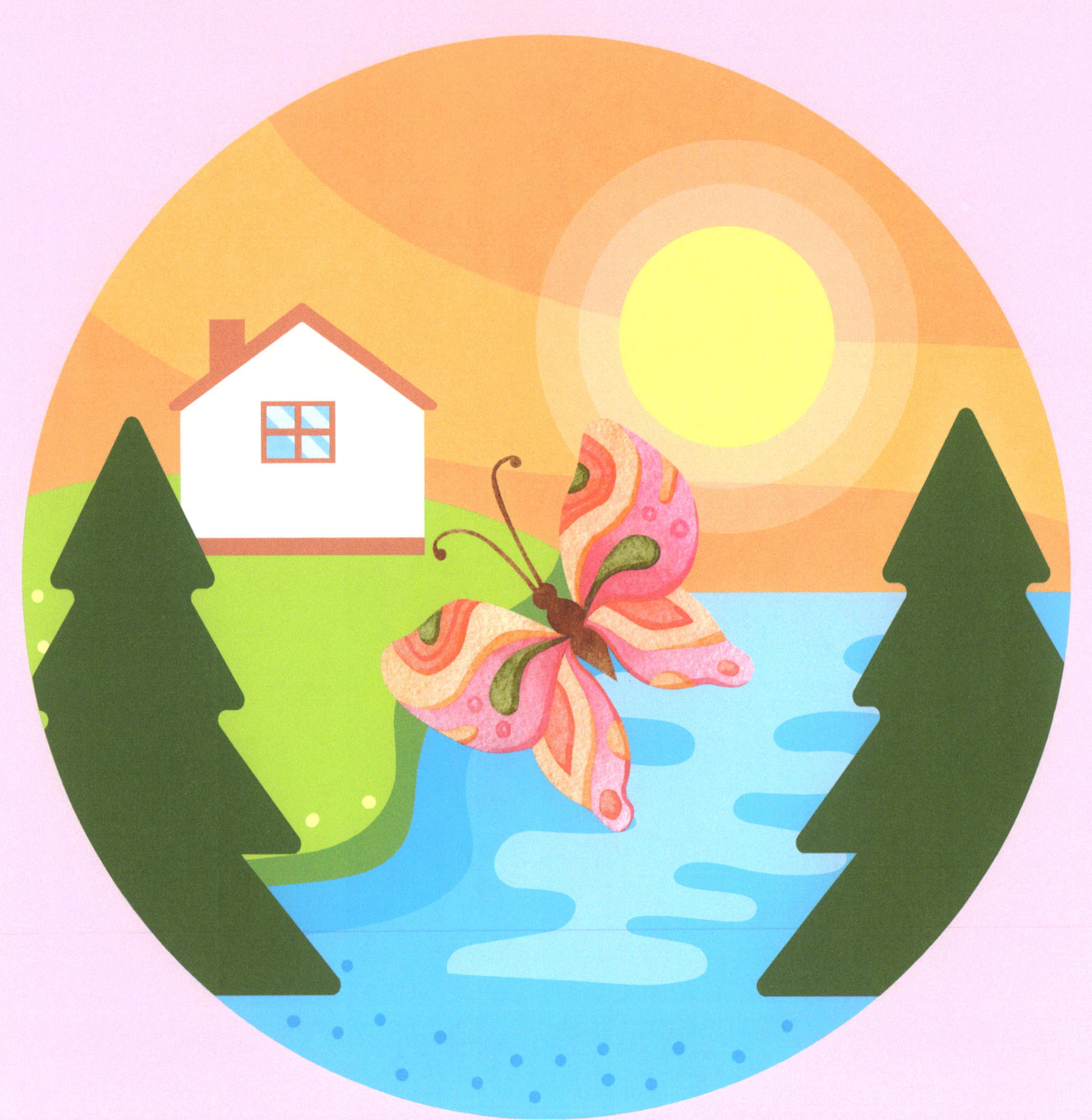

If ever you feel that your heart is sad,
Turn to family and friends to make you glad,
Just like George, you will be okay,
With love and time we will find a way.

22

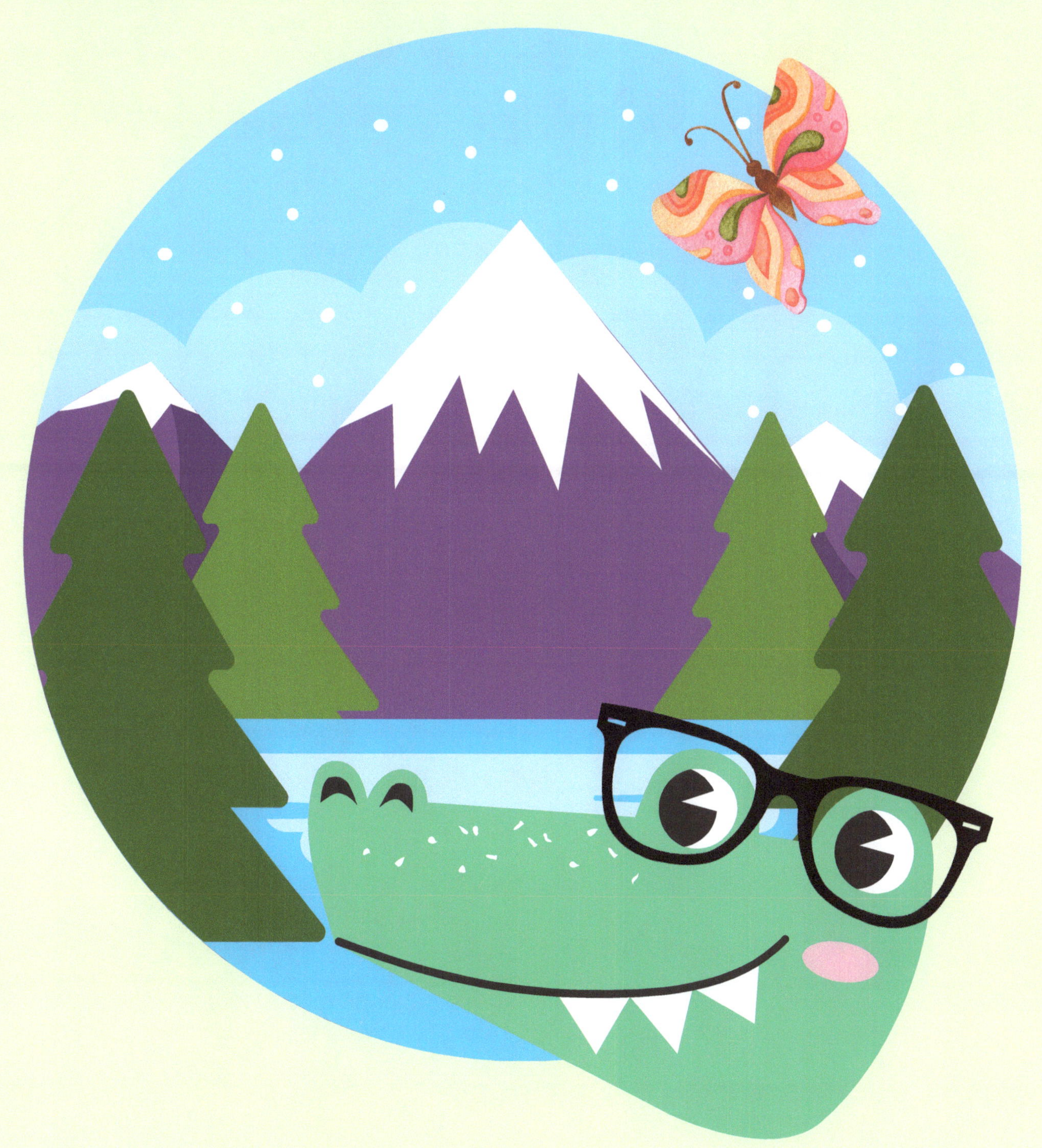

You are talented and you are strong,
You are brave as the day is long,
You are wonderfully made it is true,
You can do anything you put your mind to!

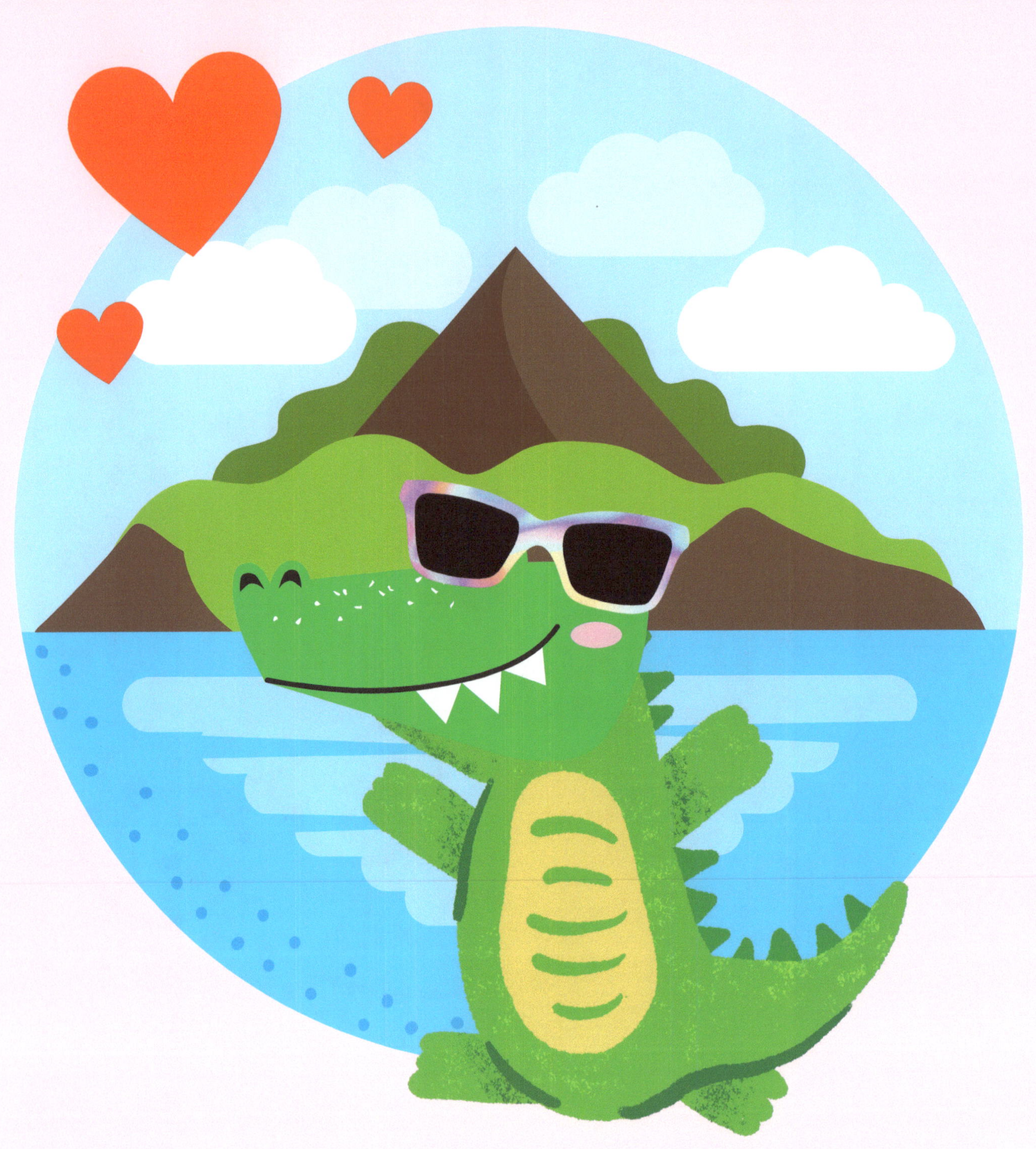

George could explore the deep blue sea,
He just saw the world a bit differently,
He could climb mountains as you can too,
Achromatopsia just makes you, you!